My Dearest Stanley,

May this book be well used! Maybe I will even do a few poses wi[...]

Enjoy[...]

D1013321

♡Beinta xoxo

bony

yoga

bony

yoga

Ryn Gargulinski

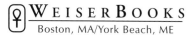
WEISERBOOKS
Boston, MA/York Beach, ME

First published in 2005 by
Red Wheel/Weiser, LLC
York Beach, ME
With offices at:
368 Congress Street
Boston, MA 02210
www.redwheelweiser.com

Copyright © 2005 Ryn Gargulinski

All rights reserved. No part of this publication may be reproduced or transmitted in any form
or by any means, electronic or mechanical, including photocopying, recording, or by any
information storage and retrieval system, without permission in writing from Red
Wheel/Weiser, LLC. Reviewers may quote brief passages.

Library of Congress Cataloging-in-Publication Data
Gargulinski, Ryn.
  Bony yoga / Ryn Gargulinski.
    p. cm.
  ISBN 1-57863-366-4 (alk. paper)
  1. Yoga—Humor. I. Title.
  PN6231.Y64G37 2005
  818.602—dc22

                            2005009604

Typeset in RotisSemiSerif by Elizabeth Wood
Printed in Canada
Friesens
12 11 10 09 08 07 06 05
 8 7 6 5 4 3 2 1

The paper used in this publication meets the minimum requirements of the American
National Standard for Information Sciences—Permanence of Paper for Printed Library
Materials Z39.48-1992 (R1997).

I tried yoga once but took off for the mall halfway through class, as I had a sudden craving for a soft pretzel and world peace.

—Terri Guillemets

contents

note to readers

Please **do** try this at home—but only with the proper instruction and preparation. This book is meant for entertainment purposes only. It does not disclose how to safely attain the positions illustrated here without breaking your neck. You'll really want to know that. Neither the author nor the publisher accepts any responsibility for injury or loss sustained in connection with the exercises and instructions herein.

☀ introduction

 Yoga's been around forever and with very good reason. Not only does it enhance your balance, rhythm, life force, and breath flow, but it leaves you with one of the most exhilarating natural highs you shall ever experience. We need not say more . . . it speaks for itself in the gentle language of peace and harmony. **Namaste.**

This guide illustrates a variety of the eighty-four yoga poses—from the basic to the advanced to the ultimately relaxed—presented to you in a thoroughly researched random order.

asana names

Do not be intimidated by the fancy schmance names of the poses. They are in Sanskrit, appropriately the oldest language on the globe. I have also provided the English names, and as you become accustomed to the lingo, you will actually be able to figure out that **asana** simply means "pose," **adho** means "facing," **mukha** is "head" and so on.

If you are one of the overly ambitious, you can even shoot to the library and get a conversation starter cassette for Sanskrit. That way you will also learn key phrases for traveling abroad like "Where's the bathroom?" and "I need a doctor."

yoga preparation

One of the most important things you can do before starting any exercise program is to buy an array of overpriced props. This type of preparation, when done correctly, will give you that warm, oozy feeling that also comes at the end of a successful workout. Most important for yoga is the sticky mat, which has that get-high rubber smell when brand-new. The mat insures that you do not slip while securing your stance and keeps the floor from penetrating your brain during inversions.

Yoga kits are also available. They usually include a mat, a foam brick, and a strap for modifying poses. Be very careful when purchasing an entire kit, for it is imperative that the mat and props come in attractive, matching colors.

A favorite CD will also enhance your workout. Any kind of music will do as long as you can balance on your head while listening to it. Movie soundtracks are recommended, especially those such as **A Clockwork Orange** and **Gangs of New York**.

Top off your props with a sexy yet functional clothing ensemble, preferably one with seams that stretch for bending and fabric that lets you breathe.

Of course, you may also take your cues from the illustrations in this book and work out naked and barefoot with no props whatsoever. It is recommended, however, you retain your skin.

Let the yoga begin!

the 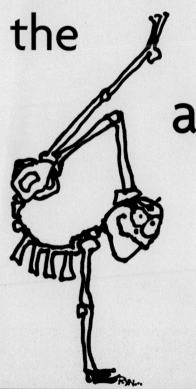 asanas

One of the most basic and fundamental poses, Mountain pose allows you to **be** that mountain. You are strong. You are stable. You are immobile. Great for confronting muggers in an alley or preventing a tumble on a crowded, roaring subway train.

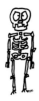

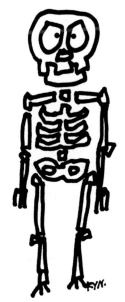

tadasana I
(mountain pose I)

You are still strong. You are still stable. You are still immobile. You are still steady on that crowded, roaring subway train—but this time you can grab an overhead handle.

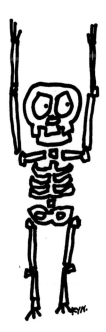

tadasana II
(mountain pose II)

The inversion poses are what makes yoga different from any other exercise. The "king" of all the poses is the all-powerful Sirsasana, or common Headstand. Not only will this pose flood you with memories of first grade gymnastics, but it will also remind you daily to view the world in a fresh, unique way. And there's no better technique for checking to see if your floor needs sweeping.

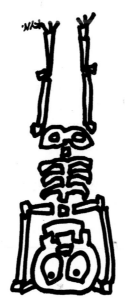

sirsasana
(headstand)

The natural complement to the king of asanas (because a king, like a president, cannot function properly without his better half) is the "queen" of asanas—Sarvangasana, or the Shoulder Stand. This pose encourages you to stop, reflect, and get grounded. It also promotes a strong neck as you will not last long with one of those floppy ones found on the bobble-headed dolls that ride in the backs of cars. This pose is ideal for sleeping in those cubicles that serve as apartments in Tokyo or getting your point across at corporate staff meetings.

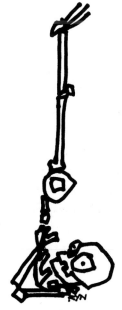

sarvangasana
(shoulder stand)

Imagine yourself the bridge—or connection—between the earthly and the sublime. You are a solid and functional bridge (like the Golden Gate, not like that structure that falls down in London). Setu Bandha Sarvangasana sets the stage for the Shoulder Stand by opening your shoulders and lengthening your back. It is also an ideal pose for wowing in the bedroom or preparing for childbirth.

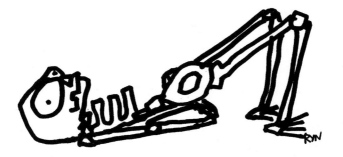

setu bandha sarvangasana
(bridge pose)

This pose is an ultimate must in any yoga regime. It stretches your entire body, from fingertips to toes. It opens your ribcage, lungs, and various organs while allowing blood to flow freshly free to your brain. Voted "Sexiest Yoga Pose" by a poll in one of those men's magazines, the Downward-Facing Dog is not recommended while wearing a bikini or in any situation in which someone has threatened to "kick your butt."

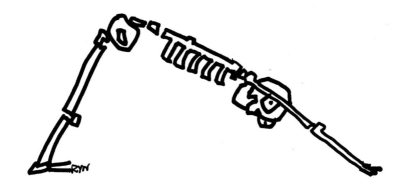

adho mukha svanasana
(downward-facing dog)

You will never again wonder how to effectively stretch your back or open your chest once you have discovered the Upward-Facing Dog. Although it appears more like an upward-facing crippled lizard, this pose is quite sexy in its own right due to the freedom and agility it helps you feel. It's also the natural choice of poses for slithering through tight spaces such as a jewelry store air duct or a basement window when you've lost your keys.

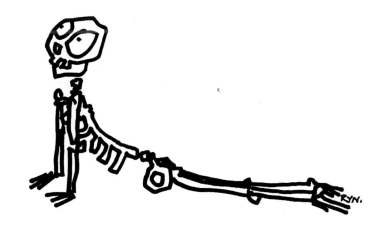

urdhva mukha svanasana
(upward-facing dog)

Similar to the Headstand, Adho Mukha Vrkasana is the pose to pick when you would rather not see how dirty your floor **really** is. Blood still rushes to your brain, internal organs still hum with life, and you are still guaranteed a massive head rush when you dismantle. The Handstand more fully develops your shoulders and forearms while ensuring your cranium does not implode—provided, of course, you do not tumble over.

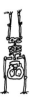

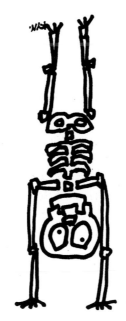

adho mukha vrkasana
(handstand)

This larch-like pose strengthens ankles and feet and steadies the knees. It's also fun to do in the park where you have the added bonus of live elm examples to emulate. Tree pose combines balance, stabilization, and centering while also looking good for photographs. Barmaids practice this pose to sneak in exercise while standing around with large trays of drinks.

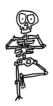

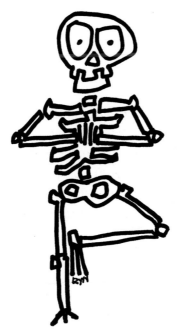

vrksasana
(tree pose)

The name alone implies the sheer power one gleans from this popular pose. One of an entire Warrior pose series, this knee-strengthening balancing act depicts a fighter poised with weapon above his head. For added effect, you may want to add a sword to your yoga workout, as long as your home has unnaturally high ceilings. This pose is also ideal for swishing ceiling spiderwebs and warming up to chop karate blocks.

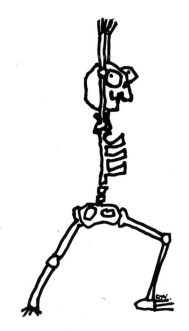

virabhadrasana I
(warrior pose I)

Perhaps the most popular and highly photographed of the Warrior poses, this stance is the epitome of the beauty of power and the power of beauty. Achilles stands like this, as do many other heroes found on Grecian urns. Fun props to add to this pose include a gilded shield and a helmet adorned with purple plume. It's also a great pose to strike at City Hall Park so small children can ask: "Mommy, what is that woman doing?"

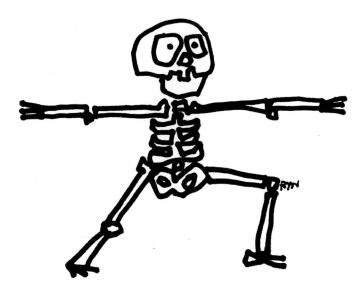

virabhadrasana II
(warrior pose II)

Rounding out the Virabhadrasana trilogy, this pose depicts the streamlined warrior shooting into battle like a bolt of lightning. Requiring exquisite balance, Warrior pose III is by far the most poised and refined. No novice fighters please. Unless, of course, you are interested in quickly learning the Losing Your Balance Warrior pose. Great for reaching over hungry shoppers in a clearance rack, this pose works well at boutiques and local malls.

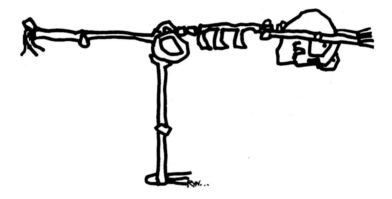

virabhadrasana III
(warrior pose III)

When done being a Warrior, it naturally follows that one should become a Hero. Virasana, they say, is terrific for increasing the quadriceps' flexibility, although the pose looks eerily like the horrendous bone-bending pose in which we sat as small children on lunchroom floors, only to be warned our legs would "freeze that way." This pose is best used while pulling weeds out of Aunt Fran's garden or watching TV (yoga videos, of course).

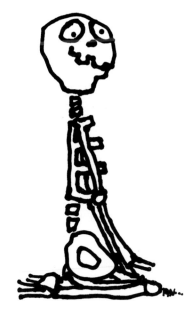

virasana
(hero pose)

Every valiant warrior needs to rest—thus another variation of the Hero pose. This one is best done after the battle, with the spoils of war—or your bloody day—strewn around you. Supta Virasana stretches the thighs, abdomen, deep hip flexors, and ankles. It also strengthens the arches in your feet to prepare you for the next rumble. Again resembling the warned-against lunchroom sprawl, it is sure to get a rise out of mothers and kindergarten teachers. Best used as preparation for being dissected by mad scientists.

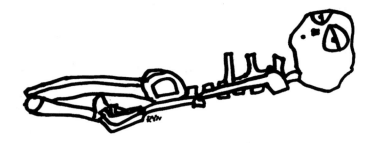

**supta virasana
(reclining hero pose)**

This is a mysterious pose, or at least mysteriously named, since it would be highly impossible for a camel to perform unless he had sunken humps. Ustrasana opens the chest, heart, and lungs while promoting freedom of the neck and healthy breathing. You will find this pose helpful for sunning that area of your neck that never seems to tan or taking a shower in a very short stall.

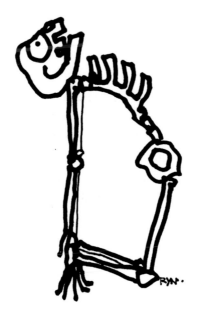

ustrasana
(camel pose)

Never mind those Japanese techno-gadgets that interpret what animals are saying when they yelp. **Becoming** that animal is the only true way to understand it. In this pose you become the feline: sexy, sleek, and arched in the back. As you slink your spine into its arch, you will know the true language of the cat. You will also get to eat raw fish, claw furniture, and spend half your waking life napping in the sun.

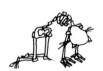

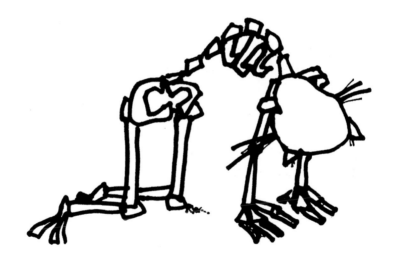

marjariasana
(cat pose)

Forearms beware! This pose demands rigorous strength, keen awareness, and, if held long enough, can promote something akin to a death wish. Great for toning the abdomen while it strengthens the wrists, arms, and spine, it challenges your balance—whether you like it or not. As the Sanskrit name so aptly conveys, this pose may make you feel like your limbs are shaking loose. A wonderful way to peer over ditches or serve as an ironing board while traveling.

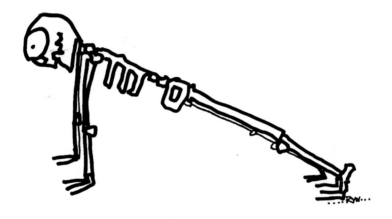

armsa falloffasana
(plank pose)

Solid, bold, and beautiful, this pose is best known for its seeming simplicity. Yet beneath its veneer of ease, Dandasana is hard at work stretching your hamstrings, strengthening your lower back, and lengthening your spine. Perfect for get-togethers in which there are not enough chairs, your willingness to sit comfortably on the floor will make you the guest they keep inviting back. You are sure to win extra points with the hostess when your straight back and extraordinary balance assure you spill no hors d'oeuvres on her new shag rug.

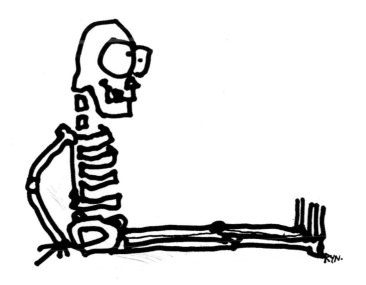

dandasana
(staff pose)

Freakish looking when done correctly, Marichyasana stretches your hamstrings and your entire backside, from your lower lumbar to your skull. It is the natural progression from Staff pose, as you remain with the solid, regal base of your lower body. You simply amend Staff by bending one leg and placing your hands behind your back, wrists clasped, enclosing your bent leg tightly between your forearm and your body. Then exhale and bend foreword. This is a wonderful way to see if you are in need of a pedicure!

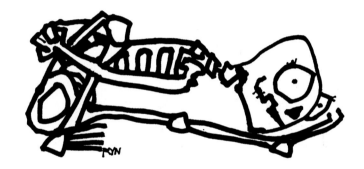

marichyasana
(one-legged forward bend)

If you want to feel a stretch that sends tingles down your side, definitely go for the Trikonasana. Aptly named for the isosceles triangle formed by your body when done correctly, you can easily experiment with different angles, as long as you don't turn it into a rectangle. Triangle pose strengthens your abdomen, legs, and back and serves as an ideal pose while babysitting. Hours of fun are sure to ensue when you ask the children "Whatever shape am I?"

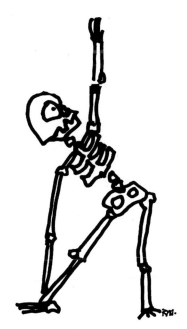

**trikonasana
(triangle pose)**

This pose, which requires supreme balance and stability, pops you open like a can of sardines. Your chest and hamstrings thrum with pleasure as you are lengthened and strengthened through the abdomen, legs, and back. Fun for the whole family, this pose insures you shall excel at Twister and never lose a game of charades.

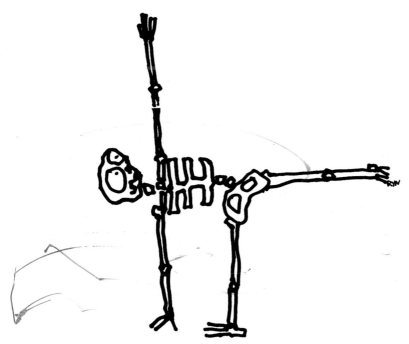

ardha chandrasana
(half moon pose)

Imagining an eagle twisting its wings and legs into something resembling an avian Twizzler is beyond the scope of most people's minds—and the pose is beyond an untrained body. Definitely for the advanced yogi, Garudasana is a wonderful way to relieve stress from the knees by lengthening the hip rotators and the ever-popular ilio-tibial band. A must in any argument you may be losing, as this pose is sure to throw your opponent off guard and cause him to forget what he is arguing about. It may also work in presidential debates.

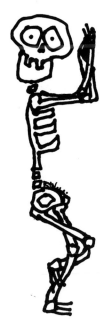

**garudasana
(eagle pose)**

Another fine pose for the stressed-out knee, Utkatasana works wonders in crowded train stations. By building up the leg, feet, and ankle muscles, it also works as a training stance for ice-skaters—exclusive of Tanya Harding. Mimes were at the forefront of the Utkatasana movement, being the first to use it openly in Western culture to mime sitting on a park bench while being trapped in an invisible box.

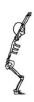

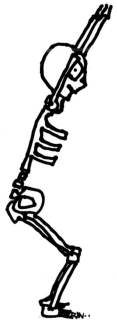

**utkatasana
(chair pose)**

This classic is an ideal way to spot-check your overall fitness factor. If you can touch your toes you are forever young— vivacious, powerful, and keen. Touching your toes is also a requirement of MENSA. Uttanasana is the base for many variations, proving its importance in the yoga scheme. Definitely a key position that works well to lengthen back muscles and lifespans.

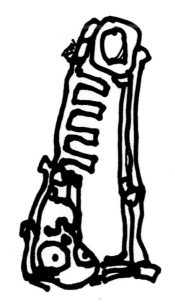

uttanasana
(standing forward bend)

Lengthen your spine, stretch your hamstrings, tie your shoes. Paschimottanasana is loaded with benefits, as evidenced by the number of Olympic athletes who swear by it. An excellent way to gently lengthen all muscles along your back, you will feel lithe and snakelike when you arise. Also works well for killing time in the ticket line while sprawled on the sidewalk outside the Sting concert.

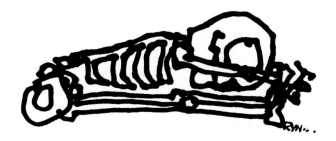

paschimottanasana
(seated forward bend)

This classic pose has a phenomenal look and feel. It also serves as an effective cure-all for the daily menaces of anxiety, irritability, and insomnia. Highly recommended for beginners and advanced students alike, Prasarita Padottanasana makes you smarter by shooting loads of blood up to your brain. It also makes the world look somewhat sensible.

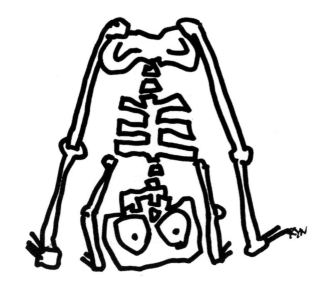

prasarita padottanasana
(wide-angle standing forward bend)

Although it may not appear to be, Halasana is deeply relaxing and sublime. It also floods the brain with blood, soothing the frazzled sympathetic nervous system. Anxiety, tension, and irritability flee as if fumigated. Your mind becomes uncluttered and serene. In fact, the only thought that may come to you is how knobby your knees are.

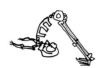

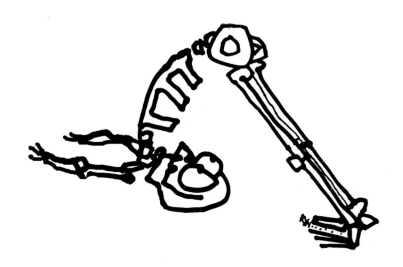

halasana
(plow pose)

Puff, puff, puff to open your chest while you stimulate your abdominal organs and stretch your neck, thighs, shoulders, groin, and often neglected psoas. Only the highly agile need attempt this deep backbend, a favorite with one-legged pigeons in Coney Island. Eka Pada Rajakapotasana was so named for the way these birds puff out their chests in seasonal mating rituals. It was also a stupendous hit in 1970s discos.

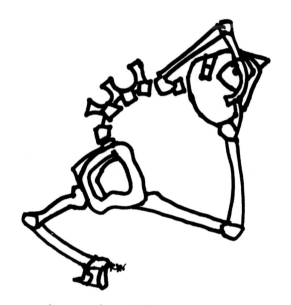

eka pada rajakapotasana
(one-legged king pigeon pose)

This gorgeous pose is sure to amaze your friends and terrify your family. Based on the ever-popular One-Legged King Pigeon pose, this inverted and modified version prevails today as one of the most amazing and impossible-looking feats of yoga. It also gives new meaning to the phrase "standing on your head." If you think this acrobatic version merely looks impossible, give it a whirl. An excellent way to impress a first date, it's the epitome of how beautiful yoga can be.

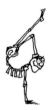

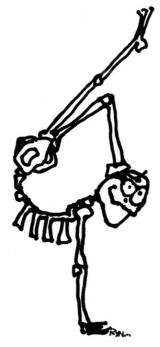

eka pada rajakapotasana (variation)
(one-legged king pigeon pose—
inverted and modified)

This advanced Staff pose builds up your arms and wrists—mainly because you are perched precariously upon them. Not a great pose for those with carpal tunnel syndrome or heavy manacles. Wonderful for finding small objects you don't want to crush—like a popped-out contact lens or your wayward pet gerbil.

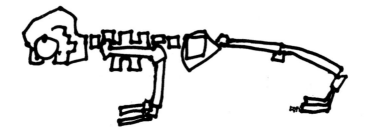

chaturanga dandasana
(four-limbed staff pose)

Rumor has it this intriguingly monikered pose actually makes your bent-up body look like a cow's face (crossed legs are the lips; bent elbows are the ears). Most humans do not see the connection, but animals have a sixth sense about such things. Cow Face pose is terrific for stretching pretty much every limb and ligament in your body. Best avoided in beef factories and during bull-mating season.

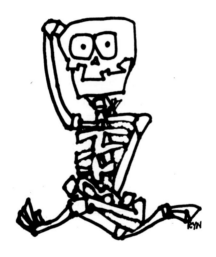

gomukhasana
(cow face pose)

Clearly one of the most industrious asanas, Supta Padangusth-asana is great for gently caressing lower inner organs and leg muscles and for stretching out pantyhose that seem to have shrunk in the wash. Men, please feel free to use a big toe prop other than pantyhose. This pose is highly rec-ommended for infertility and PMS but not one to try if plagued by diarrhea, headaches, or high blood pressure, as knowing your pantyhose no longer fit is always too stress-inducing.

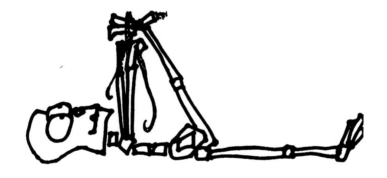

supta padangusthasana
(reclining big toe pose)

This eely asana opens the rib cage, flexes the back, and is known to induce soft hissing noises. Do not try this pose at a snake-charmer event or if you fall in a python pit. Best used for slithering into small damp places like the New York City sewer system or under your bed.

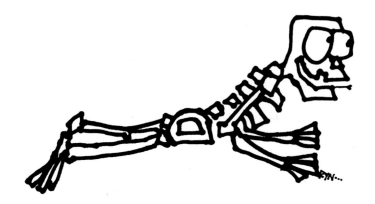

bhujangasana
(cobra pose)

One of the most advanced and gorgeous ways to arrange your body, the Crane pose strengthens your arms, elasticizes your legs and back, and firmly instills the delicate art of balance. It's the ideal pose for crossing a mud patch without soiling your shoes or leaping like a frog while drunk on eggnog.

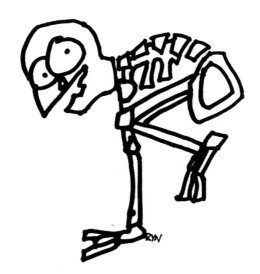

bakasana
(crane pose)

Although the ribs jut up nicely like a fish spine, experienced yogi say this pose was not named because it resembles a fish. Rather, they claim it is so named because, if you do this in water, you will float like our fine-finned friends. Until you get the hang of it, please attempt it only on land. The massive benefits of Fish pose and its variations will soon be clear—it awakens the brain and fights all diseases, including nasty bouts of guppy mouth rot.

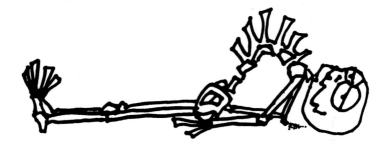

matsyasana
(fish pose)

An asana once used in Bruce Lee flicks, it stretches the limbs, stimulates the abdomen and heart, and increases poise and flexibility. It is also a perfectly intimidating way to win arguments with your annoying neighbor or a delightful way to polish and tie your shoes.

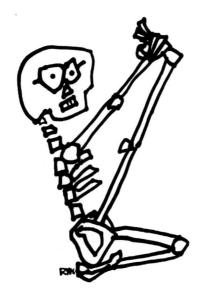

krounchasana
(heron pose)

A simple pose with many variations, the Noose pose stretches the thighs, groin, ankles, and spine while aiding digestion and elimination. This version should be done against a wall. The full pose clasps hands behind the back to resemble a noose, although it looks more like a tire swing. In either event, if this pose is done incorrectly or held for too long it may compel you to want to swing from the object for which it's named.

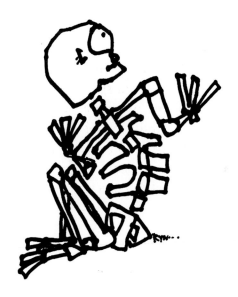

pasasana
(noose pose)

The ultimate yoga staple, this pose is depicted everywhere from holistic-healing magazine covers to modern-day bank ads that tell you to relax. And relax you it will, calming your mind, soothing your spirit, and stimulating your pelvis, spine, and abdomen. It is also an ideal pose to use if you find yourself in a small, cramped chair above a dirty floor, like in a movie theater or on a train to Shanghai or the Bronx.

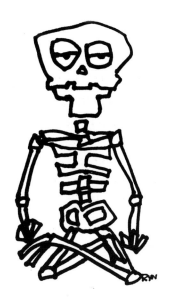

padmasana
(lotus pose)

Introduced by Hindu cheerleaders in the 8th century BC, this pose is still a staple of the modern rah-rah squad. **Hanuman** translates as "big jaws" and Hanumanasana truly takes you to limits you never knew you had. Do not try this pose if you're wearing skin-tight, leather pants; have a history of hernia; or hope to walk without bowed legs within the next six months.

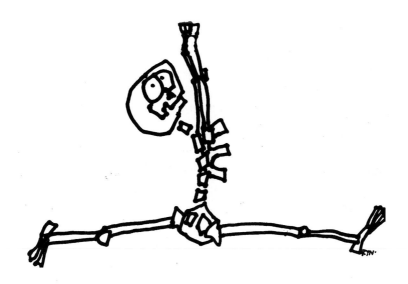

**hanumanasana
(monkey pose)**

More fun than a playground teeter-totter, the Full Boat pose strengthens the abdomen and spine, enhances digestion, and relieves stress. Frankly, there is no better way on earth to balance on your sitting bones and tailbone. Not for those with spinal injuries or excruciatingly hard, wood floors, this is a soothing way to rock a cranky toddler—or yourself—fast asleep.

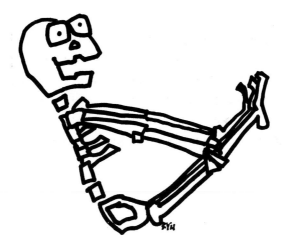

paripurna navasana
(full boat pose)

More reminiscent of a flying squirrel than a locust, this interesting pose adds might to the arms, back, buttocks, and legs. What's more, it stretches the chest and abdomen while melting stress. In some strange way, it is also known to improve posture. Perhaps it was once used as punishment for not standing up straight. It's best for body surfing the Pacific or getting out of an awkward blind date—Salabhasana guarantees your date will flee for the hills.

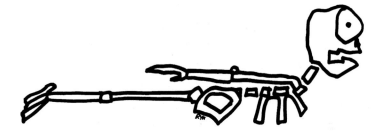

salabhasana
(locust pose)

Not surprisingly, this pose improves balance; strengthens legs, back; and neck; and assures you will always find a charming companion with whom to tango. First documented as a mating stance at an ancient Bengali ball, Natarajasana is ideal for attracting the perfect dance partner—or repelling the clod-like, clumsy ones.

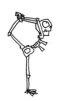

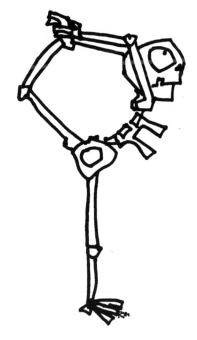

natarajasana
(lord of the dance pose)

This versatile pose elasticizes the arms and legs, stimulates the abdomen, and calms the brain. It is also a formidable pose to assume when playing Monopoly or blackjack, especially if you can use your legs to block the money or chips you are freely swiping. Upavistha Konasana also prepares you for a number of other seated yoga poses and is a great way to practice landing on thin ice.

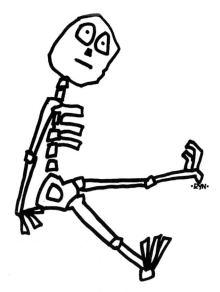

upavistha konasana
(wide angle pose)

If there were any seals that practiced yoga, you could be sure they would quickly adopt this classic pose. An excellent way to end a full yoga session, Anjali Mudra reduces stress and anxiety, calms the brain, and opens the heart to let the cosmic goodness flow in. It is also a terrific pose for saying grace before meals, posing for a snapshot you really don't want to be in, or asking your boss for a raise.

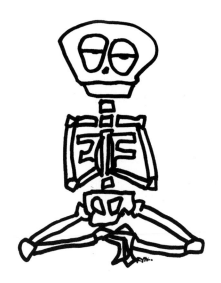

anjali mudra
(salutation seal)

This pose is best for energizing the spine and stimulating the appetite. It also awakens the digestive fires in the belly and is therefore not recommended after a heaping bowl of Texas chili. Although known to help destroy most deadly diseases, it has not proven effective in curing the common cold. Ardha Matsyendrasana is commonly seen in women's dressing rooms, as it's an excellent way to check if the jeans you're trying on are way too tight and in danger of splitting.

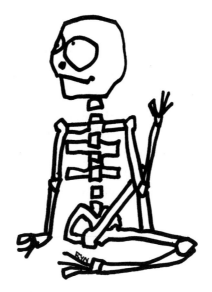

ardha matsyendrasana
(half lord of the fishes pose)

One of the three revolved standing poses, Parivrtta Parsvakon-asana stretches your arms, rib cage, neck, back, legs, and abdomen. It also increases stamina and digestion and helps clear out your intestines. This pose is recommended after a heaping bowl of Texas chili. Parivrtta Parsvakonasana has been implemented by top ice-skaters and was the highlight of a 1922 New Brunswick ice show.

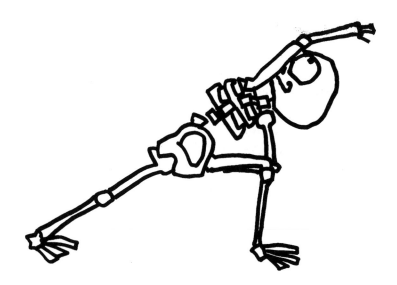

**parivrtta parsvakonasana
(revolved side angle pose)**

This comfortable pose is also known as the Cobbler pose—not because it's how you should eat apple or peach desserts, but because as it opens your groin and hips, it also allows you to fix your shoes. Baddha Konasana is one of yoga's finest poses, with myriad benefits. It stimulates major vital organs, destroys disease, and kicks fatigue right out of your bones. Best used to relax while reading trashy romance novels or watching game shows.

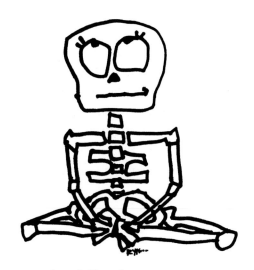

baddha konasana
(bound angle pose)

Although excellent for childbirth and PMS, men, too, will find this reclining pose useful. It relaxes the knees, hips, and groin area, relieving stress and anxiety. Best done with a bolster propped beneath your back, Supta Baddha Konasana is also great for sunning yourself on private rooftops or listening to meditation tapes. Stay in this pose for at least five minutes, or twenty-four hours if you can get away with it.

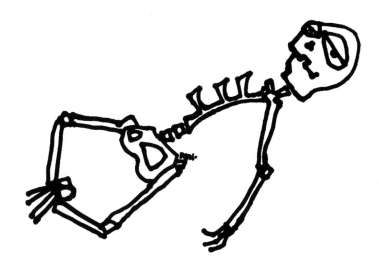

supta baddha konasana
(reclining bound angle pose)

Regress back to the womb with this cozy, embryonic position. You may even get pre-birth flashbacks provided the womb you were in smelled similar to your rubber yoga sticky mat. Balasana relieves stress in your back, arms, and neck and is especially effective after inversion poses, as it provides you a peaceful respite. Also works well for smooshing yourself into small crevices, like the cabinet under the sink in which Charles Manson hid from cops, or beneath your desk when your boss is looking for someone to blame.

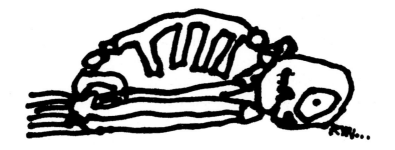

balasana
(child's pose)

Simple enough to perform nearly anywhere and comfortable enough to remain in all day, the Viparita Karani is known as the "Ultimate Relaxation" pose. To glean a supreme soothing, you need as few as five minutes, perhaps a pillow beneath your lower back, and, as the name implies, a wall. Instant tranquility will arise, smoothing frazzled nerves, easing that ball of tension in your gut, rejuvenating legs and feet, and engulfing you in an omnipresent sense of well-being. Since this pose works exceptionally well in the office (provided no loose staples litter the floor), it's a perfect way to zone out when your boss starts chewing you out for your earlier hide-under-the-desk shenanigan.

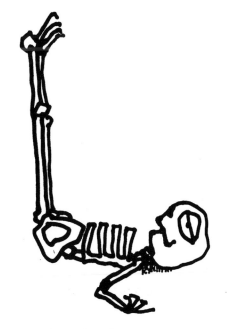

**viparita karani
(legs-up-the-wall pose)**

Perhaps the second most "Ultimate Relaxation" pose, Savasana rests every part of your overexerted body. As the name suggests, it mimics our perfect repose in death. Corpse pose is best kept for the end of a yoga session as you will become so thoroughly and limply serene you may never want to move again (and you thought Jacuzzis were heaven!). This pose was also studied by funeral directors who were not sure how to position the dead body. Symmetrical and compact, Savasana cut coffin costs in half.

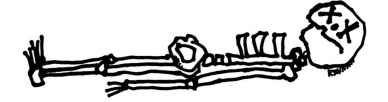

savasana
(corpse pose)

the

appendix

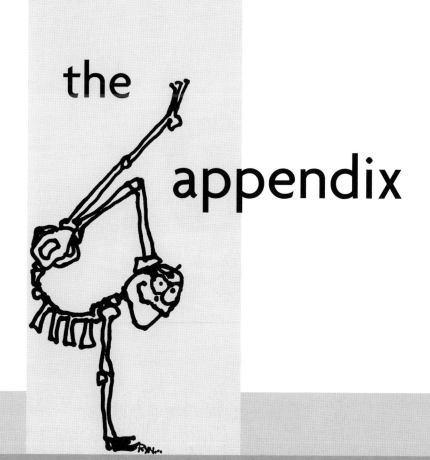

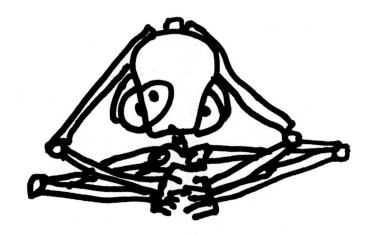

asana gone wrong . . .

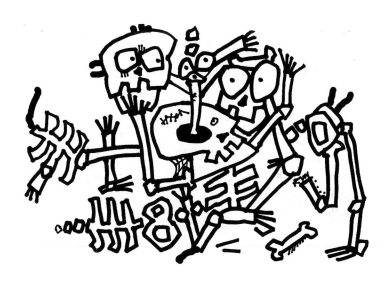

terribly wrong . . .

about the author

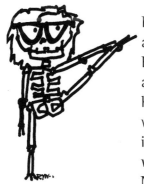

Ryn Gargulinski's main passions in life are writing and drawing. She holds a Bachelor's in Creative Writing and a Master's in English Literature, and her writing and artwork have been widely published, both online and in print, with credits including www.poetz.com, New York Newsday, New York Press, and Voices: The Journal of New York Folklore. She has also created cover illustrations for Medicinal Purposes Literary Review, The Manhattan Pet Gazette, and the Bengali poetry journal, Shabdaguchha, and has contributed her illustrated column to Brooklyn Woman newspaper and the literary Web site www.12gauge.com.

Her collections include four illustrated chapbooks, two collaborative CDs, a series of children's books, a series of illustrated humor books, and an entire line of Lucky Voodoo Dolls. To learn more about Ryn, visit her Web site at **www.ryngargulinski.com** and of course shop for her signature "RYNdustries" merchandise at **www.cafeshops.com/ryndustries**. When she's not busy creating, you can catch her doing yoga at a leafy city park or on the plains of Clovis, attempting to attain the inverted and modified Eka Pada Rajakapotasana. A recent New York transplant who misses her yoga practice on the Coney Island pier, Ryn now lives in New Mexico.

to our readers

Weiser Books, an imprint of Red Wheel/Weiser, publishes books across the entire spectrum of occult and esoteric subjects. Our mission is to publish quality books that will make a difference in people's lives without advocating any one particular path or field of study. We value the integrity, originality, and depth of knowledge of our authors.

Our readers are our most important resource, and we appreciate your input, suggestions, and ideas about what you would like to see published. Please feel free to contact us, to request our latest book catalog, or to be added to our mailing list.

Red Wheel/Weiser, LLC
P.O. Box 612
York Beach, ME 03910-0612
www.redwheelweiser.com